Caroline Flint RN RM ADM

Do Birth

A gentle guide to
labour and childbirth.

BooK Co

Published by
The Do Book Company 2013
This edition published 2023
Works in Progress Publishing Ltd
thedobook.co

To find out more about our company,
books and authors, please visit
thedobook.co or follow us **@dobookco**

A CIP catalogue record for this book is
available from the British Library

ISBN 978-1-914168-33-8

10 9 8 7 6 5 4 3 2 1

5 per cent of our proceeds from the sale
of this book is given to The DO Lectures
to help it achieve its aim of making
positive change: thedolectures.com

Cover designed by James Victore
Book designed and typeset by Ratiotype

Printed and bound by OZGraf Print on
Munken, an FSC® certified paper

MIX
Paper from
responsible sources
FSC® C163799

Contents

The basics

When you have been involved in a topic for many years – have written about it, talked about it, discussed it, lived it even – you can't help but be amazed when completely new information arrives. In 2020 – just seven short years after this book was first published – that new information about childbirth arrived. But we were in the midst of a global pandemic, so the article in medical journal *The Lancet* was hidden. No one had time to listen or take it in. Now we can take a breath and learn more.

But first let us go back to basics. The most basic fact we need to be aware of is that we are mammals. This may not seem significant, but it is of supreme importance. Mammals have been on the planet for 200 million years and during that long time they have perfected many things. Firstly, the way we grow our young is very safe. Mammals conceive inside their bodies, so the delicate embryo is protected from any harmful substances and activities, hidden away inside the female body.

The baby is nurtured inside the mother and safely grows and develops. The process of pregnancy ensures that the mother's body produces hormones which soften and stretch her uterus, her pelvic bones, her muscles, and prepare her breasts for producing milk. All very efficient.

At the right time, the woman goes into labour, which is a hormonal process aided by darkness and privacy. When I say hormones, be aware that I am talking about feelings – of love, tenderness, warmth, passion, openness, receptiveness.

All mammals labour in a similar way. They need privacy, comfort and often darkness. The labour can then progress smoothly and safely. Look at cats – well, we don't look at cats, do we? No one ever sees them in labour, they sneak away into a cupboard, under a bed or somewhere private. Dogs do the same, as do sheep, giraffes, zebra, horses. In fact, all mammals manage birth very efficiently and without much intervention. It is only occasionally that mammals need help with the birthing process.

We are living in a time of maternity investigations. A time when thousands of labouring women are traumatised, babies are distressed or worse. It is only when women are able to get to know their midwife, when there is a relationship between them, when they are friends, that the best care ensues.

We have known for 40 years that continuity of carer or getting to know your midwife ensures greater safety and satisfaction for women going through childbirth. And if you are lucky, you will be in the catchment area of the 174 areas of the UK where this form of midwifery care is practised in 2023.

Relationships are crucial to us mammals. If David Attenborough's amazing TV programmes have done nothing else, they have shown how it is the relationship between the mother and her baby which ensure the safety for the young of the species. We thrive on relationships.

We fall in love, we make love, we get pregnant and we give birth and nurture our young. If we are lucky, or we have chosen well, the other parent of the baby is there to support and love us and ensure that their child is being cared for as well as possible. Relationships matter enormously to humans, never more so than when going through one of the most intimate experiences of our lives: giving birth.

So, what were the extraordinary conclusions that came out in *The Lancet* in 2020?

The health outcomes for mothers and babies who booked for a homebirth (and I use those words advisedly because women who book for a homebirth don't necessarily end up giving birth at home) were the same as for those mothers and babies who were booked for a hospital birth, but there were big differences in other outcomes.

When women were booked for a homebirth (regardless of where they actually gave birth): [1]

— 40% fewer needed a caesarean section.

— 50% were less likely to have an instrumental delivery.

— 55% were less likely to have an episiotomy.

— 40% were less likely to have a 3rd or 4th degree tear.

— 75% were less likely to have an infection.

Looking at those figures, women were less likely to have stitches, less likely to have an episiotomy, less likely to have the trauma of forceps or ventouse. Less likely to have a surgical procedure and much less likely to have an

---

1   Source: *www.thelancet.com/journals/eclinm/article/PIIS2589-5370(20)30063-8/fulltext*

infection if they booked for a homebirth. Whether they ended up giving birth in hospital or at home! So why do we think that happened? What was going on?

Firstly, when women book for a homebirth they have, in essence, organised for a midwife to come to them at home when they go into labour. For them, there is no guessing whether they are really in labour or not, no tripping off to the hospital and being sent home because, 'You aren't in established labour, come back later when the pains are every two minutes.'

Going to hospital when you were at home – in a familiar place, open and loving because you are flooded with hormones – means that you have to interrupt that lovely atmosphere and get dressed, go outside and travel to a place with bright lights and uncomfortable furniture. It all leads to your labour stalling. Interrupted. Stopped.

But if you have booked for a homebirth, you just ring the midwife. She (I generally use the female pronoun throughout this book, but of course there are some male midwives, although at the time of writing, the majority are women) either comes immediately or listens to your voice and gives you some suggestions. You know you are on their radar. They are aware that you are in labour, and will factor that into their plans. You are immediately more confident.

Then when the midwife comes to see you the atmosphere is very different. This is your home, she is the visitor. She will ask your permission if she wants to make herself a cup of tea, or use the lavatory, or touch you. The balance of power is very different in the home. You are the boss – as you should be. She is the professional and if she is working in a homebirth team, it is highly likely that she is doing it for a reason – that she believes in women and their ability to give birth. Her response to you will be different because she has chosen to work where women are in charge, expect her to be respectful and polite, empathetic, and knowledgeable.

Be aware that emergencies do happen in childbirth, but they are actually very, very rare and with nearly all emergencies they can be predicted earlier in the labour so that there is plenty of time to transfer to hospital during the labour.

In nearly 50 years of being a midwife, I have only had to transfer one first-time mother from home to hospital in an emergency. Of course, I have transferred other first-time mothers to hospital but it has been a leisurely process, 'Would you be happier with an epidural? Shall we transfer to hospital?' or 'This labour has lasted a very, very long time, shall we go to hospital for a hormone drip to encourage things along?'

There have been transfers but they haven't been rushed. With the one emergency transfer I was able to ring the labour ward, tell the obstetrician what was happening so the theatre was all ready. The consultant obstetrician was at the front door to greet us and the transfer was smooth. The necessary caesarean was performed efficiently, and mother and baby were well cared for and healthy.

The problem we face is that, truth to tell, labour is a long, boring and tedious process. Midwives are good at long, boring and tedious – their greatest attribute is patience. Doctors, especially doctors working in hospital, are busy and less used to long, boring and tedious. They are trained to deal with emergencies. There is huge satisfaction in saving a life, performing life-changing surgery, healing broken bones, steadying an erratic heart, healing an ill patient. Doctors don't sit around waiting for things to happen, they make things happen.

This is entirely appropriate when you have cancer, heart problems, broken bones, but inappropriate for when people are dying or in labour. Both situations are served best by watchful support, encouragement and patience. This is why midwives have better results than doctors in childbirth and why hospital is so unsatisfactory if the person is dying. They need peace and quiet, gentle voices, softness and warmth and, above all, patience! I'm sorry to lump labour and dying together but they are similar processes and many women recognise this when they are in labour: it is as if the curtain between one world and the next is slightly open, flapping in the breeze.

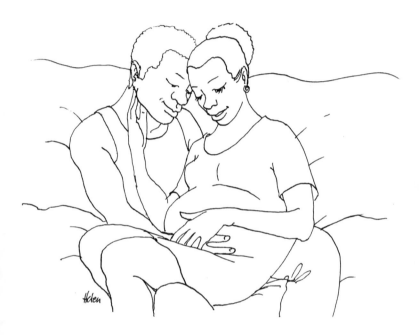

The beginning

Birth is the beginning, the very beginning. It is the start of a new life: for your baby, for you and for your partner.

For your baby, birth is the beginning of independent life. For you, it is the beginning of becoming a mother. For your partner, the beginning of becoming a parent. For all of you, birth is the beginning of becoming a family.

A gentle birth, where the baby is welcomed with tenderness, soft voices, dim lights and gentle handling, tells the baby that they are welcome in the world, that their parents are pleased to see them and that the world is a kind and loving place. A brutal entry into the world, where the baby is pulled out of their mother's body, accompanied by loud voices and bright lights, and then rubbed with a rough towel, teaches this oh-so-sensitive baby that the world is a tough place where they may not always be welcome. How we handle a new baby is so very important.

This human being has spent their life so far in utter bliss: constantly cuddled in the mother's soft, undulating uterus and fed all the time through the umbilical cord via the placenta.

Think what it is like for your baby snuggled in your uterus, sucking up the sweet amniotic fluid whenever they fancy a drink. Your amniotic fluid has a completely unique taste that teaches your baby what you smell like – which is why all newborn mammals can identify their mother by smell. When your baby emerges into the world, they recognise this familiar smell. They also hear your familiar, comforting voice and your partner's warming tones. Instead of being stroked by the soft uterus, they are stroked by your soft, loving hands, kissed by your tender lips, gently murmured to and surrounded by laughter and joy. What a lovely welcome; what a wonderful beginning.

As a practising midwife, I have been welcoming babies into the world for nearly 50 years and I couldn't have wished for a better job. The purpose of this book is to help you to have a birth that you can look back on with great joy; and to give birth in a place where you feel safe and comfortable. I may not be able to be there in person, but I hope that this book is the next best thing!

You are setting out on the most exciting, exhilarating and yet the most exhausting and gruelling experience of your life. It is an experience that you will remember with great clarity until you are a very old woman. Ask any granny about the birth of her child (especially the birth of her first child), and she will be able to give you a blow-by-blow account of the birth of Fred 52 years ago, or Marilyn 48 years ago, or Debbie 36 years ago. The memory of the birth of her first baby will be clearer than the memory of her husband's proposal, her wedding day, getting her degree or any of the other important occasions during her life. The birth of a child, particularly of a first child, is probably the most important experience of our lives.

None of us can know what sort of labour we are going to have until we are in it. Birth is so extraordinarily variable. Some births are fine, easy, not very painful and fairly quick. Other births are absolutely ghastly – long, painful, simply horrible. Thank goodness for modern pain-relieving methods.

What sort of labour do you envisage? The easy type? Or do you anticipate that your labour will be difficult? Can you influence how labour goes, or is it completely out of your hands? How exactly can you prepare?

If you have a straightforward first pregnancy and would like to remain at home when you go into labour, then there is no reason why you shouldn't stay at home for the entire labour and birth. During my career, I have come to believe that having your baby in a place where you feel comfortable and uninhibited – a familiar, welcoming place – can make all the difference to your labour and your baby's entry into the world.

Your home is a private place, it is quiet; home is clean with very few nasty germs. Home is soft and comfortable; it is where you feel safe and where you make love to your partner – in turn triggering the release of the hormone oxytocin – and labour is the time to release more oxytocin than ever before (more on that later!).

During the course of this book, I'll explain how to arrange to have your baby at home; what you can expect during labour and immediately afterwards; and how to bond with your baby during those tricky first weeks.

But first and foremost, my advice is to book a homebirth. By doing this, you are arranging for a midwife to come to your home when you are in labour and to stay with you throughout labour. The care you will receive is more personal and is focused completely on you: you won't feel that you are being pushed along a conveyor belt of generic care. If, when the time comes, you find labour far more challenging than you had anticipated, you can always change your mind and ask to be transferred to hospital.

This book is for everyone who wants to have their baby at home. It is also for those who want to stay at home as long as possible during labour. And lastly, it is for those who want to know how to make a hospital birth as familiar, gentle and homely as possible.

1
Where should I have my baby?

Homebirth is fairly unusual these days, but this hasn't always been the case. Think about almost every genius you have ever heard of and the likelihood is that they will have been born at home – Mozart, Beethoven, Einstein, Elgar. They were all born in their mother's home, attended by a midwife or female helper, comfortably and without ceremony. Very little drama, just a baby slipping into the world.

When I had my first baby, 30 per cent of babies were born at home. Today it's as little as 2 per cent. I had no intention of having my first baby at home. I was a modern woman, and modern women had their babies in hospital. Then I discovered an unpalatable truth – that men weren't allowed in the labour ward. At that time, they were meant to pace up and down outside or sit in the pub nursing a pint. I realised that I needed my husband Giles there with me. Who else could I swear at? Who else loved me above all others and would keep me safe? Who else smelt comforting and familiar? Who else would stroke me and comfort me when I was in pain? So, after much deliberation, I decided to have my first baby at home.

That decision led me to the most wondrous experience of my life. It was a painful and tedious process, sweaty, tearful and pukey; yet also powerful, amazing and ecstatic. An experience that I will remember with joy, gratitude and absolute clarity until the day I die. Not a single detail is forgotten, and each year on my son's birthday, I relive the day of his birth with pleasure and affection. Affection for the lovely midwife – working there on her own; affection for my lovely husband – completely blown away by the experience; and affection for my lovely son – who has become such a wonderful husband and father himself.

The labour and birth of our first babies is a time of heightened awareness, and the memories become part of who we are and the women we become. Therefore it is really important to make the experience as good as possible so it becomes a pleasant memory. If you live on a remote island or at the top of an inaccessible mountain and miles away from a hospital, it is probably not a good idea to have a homebirth for your first child. However, if you live in an urban environment, with a hospital within easy reach, it is a perfectly reasonable decision to book a homebirth with your local midwives or with an independent midwife.

We often hear that there is a shortage of midwives, but few people explore the reasons why. We are talking about the most exciting and stimulating job in the world, a job full of variety and hope, a job where you see a miracle happen almost on a daily basis. What's not to love? Midwives are paid a decent amount (nothing like bankers' huge bonuses, but a sensible and good amount).

There is a shortage of midwives because as women are encouraged to have their babies in hospital, so midwives are brought into hospitals. There, many are subjected to rules, regulations and guidelines that go against their deepest instincts and prevent them from practising as true midwives. They do their best, they try hard to protect women from the prevailing philosophy of 'What if something happens?', 'What if something goes wrong?' In spite of themselves, they are caught up in the drama of 'a disaster waiting to happen'. And because women in labour are extremely sensitive to atmosphere, the 'disaster waiting to happen' often becomes the disaster that happens. Hence the huge number of women who say, 'Thank goodness I didn't have my baby at home.' Sometimes I want to cry! It is such nonsense. Just as much a nonsense as the caesarean section rate in the city in which I live.

London is one of the richest cities in the world; even during a recession people in London are better off and better fed than almost anywhere else. Women are well nourished and educated. They have babies that they choose to have and access to excellent medical facilities. There are fewer women with high-risk pregnancies in the developed world at the moment than in the whole history of humankind. Yet nearly 50 per cent of women having babies for the first time in London hospitals end up having a caesarean section.

In my view, there has been an erroneous insistence from the medical profession that the birth of a woman's first child should be in hospital. Then, once the woman's body has 'proved itself', a homebirth could be a possibility for her second child. I have been a midwife for 47 years. During that period I have attended hundreds of homebirths and births in non-medicalised, midwife-led birth centres and I have had one obstetric emergency with a woman having a first baby: only once when I have had to call an ambulance, when I had to ring the nearest labour ward and say, 'We are coming in, cord prolapse at full dilatation. Please get the theatre ready.' (Mother and baby were both fine after a caesarean section.) Now I wish I could say to you that this low statistic is because I am a brilliant midwife, but to be honest, I can't. I am a bog-standard midwife – patient, good at sitting and waiting for long periods, encouraging and upbeat. The reason that I have had so few emergencies is because first labours are usually extremely safe and straightforward.

There is a greater likelihood of transferring to hospital with a first labour, but that is usually because the labour has lasted for days. First labours are very predictable; they meander on with contractions coming regularly and cervical dilatation occurring gradually. The midwife can usually judge that there is time to pop out and do a visit, that she can go home for a snooze, set her alarm for four hours later and come back. If a transfer to hospital is contemplated, it can normally be done in a leisurely fashion: 'Now, Maddy, you have been in labour for nearly three days. It is time to think about going to hospital for an intravenous drip of syntocinon (synthetic oxytocin) to help your contractions become more effective, and maybe a nice epidural. Please think about it over the next couple of hours.'

So where should you have your baby?

We are mammals, like dogs, cats, horses, deer, pigs and sheep. Like all other mammals, we are surprisingly good at giving birth. We nourish and cherish our babies inside our bodies until they are ready to emerge. We go into labour spontaneously and labour over a few days. It is perfectly normal for a first labour to last around 24–48 hours.

Like all mammals, we are very instinctive. We always adopt physiologically favourable positions during labour, which enable our babies in-utero to be well oxygenated and help them to move down the birth canal. Given a choice, women rarely lie down in labour. They lean, they stand, they kneel forwards, they squat in the bath or they sit on the lavatory.

Think about other mammals in labour. The domestic dog goes underneath your bed, makes herself a little nest with your old jumper and a soft cloth and sits there in private. Your domestic cat chooses the airing cupboard or somewhere where she can be private and not overlooked. Cows choose the corner of the field, quite apart from the rest of the herd. Horses find a dark corner of the stable where they can hide away. As mammals, we need privacy during labour. We also need darkness. During 47 years of being on call as a midwife, I have been called during daylight hours on just 15 occasions.

The dark hides us and gives us more privacy. And it's also in darkness that we release more of the hormone oxytocin, the hormone that stimulates our uteruses to contract and thus open the cervix during labour. Oxytocin is exactly the same hormone that we release when making love and having an orgasm, often done in darkness too. We need to consider childbirth as part of our sex lives, and plan our venue accordingly. Personally I can't imagine becoming sexually aroused in a brightly lit hospital, can you?

Like dolphins and whales who may be assisted during birth by a 'midwife' dolphin or whale, we are mammals who often choose to have an expert with us to help and guide us. How will you know otherwise that you are in labour? You may be having uterine contractions every 10 minutes, but are you actually in labour? Or is this false labour, or the latent phase of labour?

So, how do you make sure that you have this expert by your side? One route is to pay for an independent or freelance midwife to attend to you throughout your labour and birth. They may also help look after you and your baby during the early weeks. Alternatively, you can employ a doula – someone who provides practical, emotional, but non-medical, support during pregnancy, childbirth and early parenthood. Or, if you live in the UK, you can get all this for free with the NHS by booking for a homebirth.

When you book for a homebirth, you don't necessarily give birth at home – you can transfer to hospital at any stage. You may decide that you need an epidural, or you may want to go into hospital because you feel safer there or because you are getting bored and think that a change of scene will accelerate things. Everything is flexible. However, being at home during labour is one of the best ways to ensure that you are looked after beautifully.

You will be attended throughout established labour by one midwife who will remain with you, and a second midwife who will usually join her for the actual birth. Some women worry that they may be depriving someone more needy of a midwife's attention. My response is that this is the most important experience of your life, so it's essential to make sure it is as good as possible. Being a mother is a demanding and responsible 24/7 job, so it's best to feel as strong, invincible and competent as possible when you begin that journey. Over the years I have seen women feel this way much more with homebirths than with hospital births.

I feel that I should make my position on hospitals clear. As an ex-nurse I love hospitals. My husband says that I am like a horse scenting water when I enter them; he expects me to rush over to someone's bed to plump up their pillows! Hospitals are beautifully and specifically designed for treating ill people. Plenty of light needs to be cast on the patient who lies at a height that everyone can access. This is brilliant for strokes, heart attacks, surgery, cancer, pneumonia, the list goes on, but not appropriate for a mammal needing privacy, darkness and soft comforts.

The same applies to doctors being involved in childbirth. Doctors are trained to think that childbirth is a dangerous time. They are men and women of action. We expect a doctor to do something when we are ill or needing surgery. If I ever have a heart attack, I hope the nearest doctor will do something, and not just pat my hand anxiously and say, 'Caroline, I hope you don't die.' We expect doctors to act, which is why their care can be so counter-intuitive to childbirth. They are not trained to be patient, they are doers. So they speed up slow labours, start up late ones, use ventouse and forceps to bring out the baby or carry out a caesarean section. All of these actions can be beneficial in a very slow labour, or in a labour in which mother and/or baby need medical help. However, so many doctors find it almost impossible not to intervene unnecessarily: they must always be doing something to help things along.

When midwives are experienced and strong, they keep doctors away from women in normal labour. They guard her privacy and allow the doctor in only when they are needed: when action is needed. The tragedy of modern times is that doctors don't see that their presence is an intervention in itself.

Let's look at this another way. Just imagine that you say to your partner or to your mum, 'I'm going to the loo to do a poo,' and their immediate reaction is, 'Okay, I'll call the doctor. They wanted to be here to make sure that everything goes smoothly.' No sooner do you sit on the loo seat than the door opens and in strides your doctor.

'Hi, Samantha, just wanted to come over when you defecated in case of an emergency. Just ignore me, I'll sit quietly on the laundry basket and then leap into action if anything goes wrong.' They sit there and you become more and more embarrassed. You try to hold back any unsociable noises and to smooth your skirt over your thighs so they can't see anything. Basically, you are trying to do a poo without anyone seeing and without making a sound.

Next the doctor says, 'Samantha, I can't really see what is going on, do you mind lying on a bed? Don't worry about any mess, we'll put some wadding under your bottom to catch anything.' You lie on the bed and they watch you with great concentration. Next, your mum comes to see what is going on and whether she can help. You think you will die of embarrassment. I won't go on, but your simple act of doing a poo will likely end up with you needing enemas, suppositories, all sorts of help. 'Help' for a perfectly normal everyday experience, which you could have accomplished on your own. Get my meaning?

At home, your environment is private and secure: no one can enter unless you let them. You have created your home to suit your tastes, with comfortable furnishings and ambient lighting. Your kitchen cupboards are stocked with things that you like to eat. You may have anchovy paste for your toast, or marmalade, or peanut butter, grapefruit

squash or Lapsang Souchong tea. Your home smells of
you and your partner – a comforting and familiar smell.
Above all, your home is clean. It is unlikely that there will
be any infectious bacteria here – no MRSA or C. difficile. It
is a gentle and undemanding environment. Here you can
give birth to your child and start your new life together
in privacy, not overlooked or pressured to move on to the
busy postnatal ward to make way for someone else.

After the birth, you will snuggle in bed with your
beloved partner and gaze at your baby, telling each other
how very clever you are – lovely, fragrant, joyful and
transcendant.

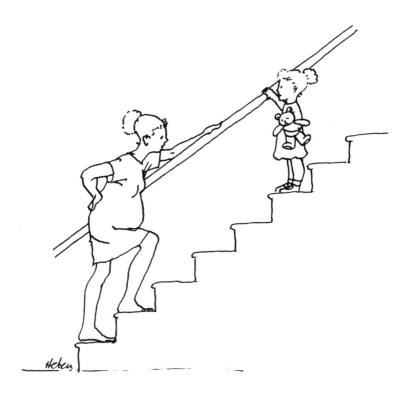

2
Making preparations

In practical terms, to arrange to have your baby at home, you need to contact the community midwives in your area and ask them to book you in for a homebirth.

It is a fairly straightforward procedure. You can discuss it with the midwife at your booking-in appointment, or simply ring the community midwives directly. In some areas, you email the homebirth team – every area is different. It is unlikely, though, that your doctor will know what you should do as this is not their area of expertise. If you can't locate the number for the community midwives in your area, ring your local maternity hospital and ask them for it. If you have no response, contact the Head of Midwifery at your local maternity hospital. You may want to follow up your phone call with a letter so that you have a written record that you requested a homebirth.

Once you have booked yourself in for a homebirth, you will be allocated a midwife who will start to visit you regularly at home. The quality of antenatal care will improve because it is more personal. She will perform all your antenatal checks, such as taking your blood pressure and doing urine tests. She will also feel your tummy to see how well your baby is growing. She will tell you what you need to do to get ready for the birth and will give you a number to ring when you think you are in labour. When your due date approaches, she will bring all the things she will need for the birth and drop them off at your home.

Things your midwife will need

Discuss with your midwife what she will bring to the birth and what you will need to provide. Usually your midwife will turn up with a limited amount of equipment which might include:

— **gas and air** (Entonox) for pain relief
— **sterilised instruments**
— **medical gloves**
— **kitchen roll**
— **absorbent pads** to cover the floor and/or bed
— **a hand-held mirror** to help see what is going on if you are in an inaccessible position
— **a torch** in case you prefer to labour in the dark

If your labour goes on for a long time, your midwife will get hungry. While a four-course gourmet meal is not expected, it's a good idea to have stock items in your cupboard such as tea, coffee, bread, cake or – a popular choice – chocolate biscuits. Make sure you have enough milk for cereals and hot drinks. Check, too, if your midwife has any specific food or drink requirements. Some midwives I know ask for a certain type of cheese to snack on during the labour, others like goats' milk for their tea; ask her what would make her more comfortable during the party.

If you are worried about your flooring, discuss this with your midwife too. Usually midwives bring absorbent pads to cover the floor during a homebirth. Personally I avoid plastic sheeting for the floor, as if it gets wet, it is very slippery and can be lethal!

It's a good idea to have a spare torch to hand. Your midwife may bring her own in anticipation of working in a dark room, but it's useful to have one in reserve as our torches often run out of batteries or get 'drowned' if they fall in a birth pool.

A spare mirror is also useful. At a birth I recently attended, I was unable to see a thing at one point. The husband and wife were completely entwined and my mirror was in the bedroom down the corridor – at that particular stage of the labour I couldn't leave long enough to retrieve it!

Things you will need in labour

It's important to keep your blood sugar levels stable during labour. If you are hungry, not only might you become more grumpy, tearful, shaky or down, but hunger can also make it harder to cope with pain. Your partner can encourage you to snack regularly.

Stock up on energy foods, such as honey, that you can add to fruit teas or on top of toast. Chocolate is good, as are muesli bars and bowls of cereal. Glucose tablets and glucose drinks are helpful, too, especially if you feel nauseous or vomit during labour and can't stomach the thought of eating food.

And make sure you drink plenty of fluids too. Have to hand small refillable bottles of water that have a spout top you can suck from. These are incredibly useful as you can drink from them at any angle during labour and they don't spill when left on a bed or the floor. Squash is an easy way to replenish your blood sugar levels; avoid ones that say 'no added sugar'. Pink grapefruit, lemon or orange barley are all refreshing. Coca-Cola and apple juice are popular in labour too.

Your uterus is the biggest muscle in the human body, and it contracts strongly every 5–10 minutes for 24–48 hours in a first labour, depleting your body of energy and lowering your blood sugar. So munch your way gently through labour to give yourself the energy you'll need to keep going.

You will also need:

— **Large sanitary towels** – maternity pads or night-time pads.
— **A couple of rolls of cotton wool**
— **Spare kitchen rolls**
— **A couple of small, old towels** – these are for when you wash after the birth. Smallish is best and old is even better (more absorbent). You are likely to be bleeding for the first 24 hours after the birth and are bound to get blood on your towel, so it's best to use one that can be thrown away afterwards.
— **A large plastic bowl** – this can be used to keep water in for washing or cooling you down, or for you to be sick into.
— **A couple of cotton flannels (washcloths)** – these can be soaked and used to soothe your sweaty brow or cool your hot neck.
— For pain relief during labour, it is well worth buying **tablets that are a mixture of paracetamol 500 mg and codeine approx. 8 mg**. They are called different names according to the pharmacy that produce them. These really help you to cope with the pain. Your doctor may prescribe pure codeine tablets if you are booked

for a homebirth, which are even stronger than the paracetamol and codeine mix.

— **Music or relaxation tapes**
— **A camera** to record these most precious moments. You can always delete ones afterwards that you don't like, but these moments are unique. Children love seeing the very first images of themselves.

Things your baby will need:

— **A packet of disposable nappies** – buy the smallest size for newborns. I suggest that you use disposables during the first six weeks when life is so demanding. You can switch to reusable nappies after that if you wish.
— **A packet of nappy wipes** (unscented).
— **A first outfit** – a cotton vest and all-in-one babygro.
— **A soft blanket** – to wrap your baby in.
— If you are having a summer baby, **a cooling fan** is helpful, although it's best not to leave this on for long or aim it directly at the baby.

What to wear during labour

During labour, choose clothing that is loose and cool and that's easy to move around in. An old, large, clean T-shirt with shorts or tracksuit bottoms is ideal. Avoid any fussy clothing. It is likely that your feet will be swollen, so flip-flops are a sensible choice.

Your partner also needs comfortable and cool clothing as they may get hot, sweaty and tired.

Knickers are necessary to keep your sanitary towel in place after the birth. Again, wear old ones that you don't mind throwing away afterwards. Granny knickers or bikini briefs are best (rather than G-strings!) or disposable knickers. Avoid paper disposable knickers as these tend to tear or cut into you.

The birthing pool

Being able to luxuriate in a deep pool of water can make a magical difference to labour. If you are planning to have your baby at home, I would strongly advise that you get a birthing pool. Even if you are not anticipating giving birth at home, it is still worth hiring or buying one for the early stages of labour. And if you are heavily pregnant during the hot summer months, a birthing pool can be a godsend. Cooling and invigorating, you can splosh around in it feeling supported and nimble. Lovely!

Being submerged in warm water soothes muscles and increases relaxation, which helps to make the pain much more manageable. The water also makes you more buoyant and able to take up the most extraordinary positions, thus opening your pelvis in a way that you never could on dry land. Being in a deep pool enhances your feeling of privacy, too, enabling you to relax and release more oxytocin. It is unusual (but not impossible) for partners to get in the pool with you. If your partner is getting in, they need to decide what they want to wear, or not wear, in the pool: a swimming costume/trunks is fairly standard.

You can buy or rent a birthing pool. You can also try eBay for a second-hand one. Some midwives have a pool that they can bring, so it is worth asking before you invest in one.

It is important to set up the pool well before your due date. There is nothing worse than everyone rushing round trying to fill a mammoth pool with water at the right temperature while the mum-to-be is in the throes of labour.

I would advise that you set the pool up at 36 weeks, about a month before your due date. A birthing pool is big and takes up a lot of room, so the best place for it is in a corner of the room, which is also where the floor is strongest as the joists overlap. Your midwife will have access on two sides, which is sufficient.

Decide on which room you want to be in. Ideally, choose one that is relatively private and can be made fairly dark with window blinds or curtains.

Once your pool is constructed, fill it. Yes, today! You need to ensure that your hosepipe is long enough for both filling and emptying the pool. Not only do you need to check on the hose length, but you also need to ensure that you have the right adaptors to fit on your taps. This exercise is also useful so you know how long filling your pool takes.

First, fill the pool with a good inch of cold water – this ensures that when the hot water is added less steam is generated – then add hot and cold water as you wish. Once your pool is full, try it out so you get used to the feel of it and how the world looks from it before you are in labour. Taking a trial dip helps you work out if, say, you need a small towel made into a head rest, a coffee table close at hand for your water bottle – or anything else you might need.

You can empty the pool by pump into the bath or lavatory. You can also empty the pool by syphonage if it is on a slightly higher level than the place you are emptying it into, such as the garden or a drain.

If you are having a hospital birth, or you are transferred to hospital during labour, most hospitals have birthing pools that you can use. You just have to hope that there isn't already someone in it!

3
The baby is coming!

You are all set up for labour. Your midwife's contact number is to hand; old, but clean, towels are at the ready; and your food and drinks cupboards are well stocked. You are ready and waiting. So what do you do when your due date comes and goes? Is there anything you can do to help labour start?

The substance that is thought to help labour start is prostaglandin. The good news is that there is plenty of prostaglandin in semen. So, although not proven, one possible way to help your baby on their way is to make love at every opportunity. In fact, most loving encounters with your partner will trigger the release of oxytocin, which encourages your uterus to contract – even if these contractions are only of the Braxton Hicks muscle-flexing type.

Some people recommend eating six dates every day from 36 weeks to stop you going too overdue, or drinking raspberry leaf tea from around 32 weeks, which is thought to prime your uterus for labour.

If you do go overdue, this can mean simply that your body is taking longer than the recommended 40 weeks to make a baby. From a homebirth perspective, the only problem with going overdue is that your midwife will be put under pressure to bring you into hospital for an induction. This is when your labour is started artificially – either by a small pill placed under your tongue or a gel put around your cervix. Once you have been induced, a homebirth is ruled out as you will need regular electronic monitoring and so will have to stay in hospital until your baby is born. Some hospitals have a policy to induce at 42 weeks, others at 40 weeks plus 10 days. You can always negotiate with the doctors. If you are happy with being pregnant and would rather wait until your baby is ready to come out, you can make that decision, but the doctors and midwives will tell you why they are suggesting an induction. It is worth reading *cochrane.org* and looking at the research about prolonged pregnancy, then you can make up your own mind. It is clear that some women take longer than others to be ready to give birth. Normal is from 36–42 weeks.

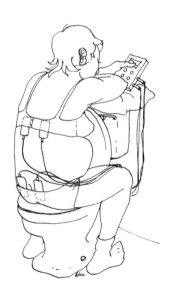

The latent phase of labour or 'pre-labour'

Labour starts when you begin to have contractions of your uterus. This is a feeling of dragging deep inside your body, very low in your abdomen or back. It is a very tense contraction of your muscle accompanied by cramping sensations, a bit like a period pain. These contractions come and go, and when they are not there, they are not there – no pain, no discomfort.

So you may be having contractions, but are you actually in labour? It is possible that you are in the latent phase of labour, or 'pre-labour'. This is when you have painful and fairly regular dragging sensations in your lower abdomen, but your cervix is not yet ready to dilate. These contractions may keep you awake at night and demoralise you – because when you call the midwife and she examines you vaginally you may not have dilated at all! The contractions can feel sharp because as the cervix is not dilating, you are not producing endorphins to help you. This 'pre-labour' stage is where a TENS machine can come into its own.

TENS is short for Transcutaneous Electrical Nerve Stimulation. It is a small, portable, battery-operated box with wires attached to four pads that you stick on to your back – your lower back where the dimples in your bottom are, and slightly higher, roughly where your bra strap sits (see picture). The pads transmit regular electrical pulses, like small electrical shocks, that are thought to block pain signals and appear to increase your endorphin production. You control the strength and frequency of the pulses, making them faster or slower, stronger or weaker, as you wish. It's useful to have a spare set of pads, particularly if you have self-stick ones, which can get messy during a long labour as paper gets stuck to them or they fold over on themselves and fail to stick to you. Either way, a TENS machine is a very popular method of pain relief during this early phase. If you would rather not have the added cost of buying one, they are available to hire.

The other great aid during this very frustrating phase of labour is alcohol. While I don't recommend drinking during pregnancy, a glass of wine at this stage to help you relax is okay. Couple this with a nice soak in the bath (take the TENS pads off for this!) and you'll start to feel much more comfortable.

If you feel too restless to lie in a bath, move around instead. This is a good way to keep your labour progressing and to help dull the pain. Keep nourished with your sugar-rich snacks and hydrated with plenty to drink. Pass urine regularly, too, as a full bladder can obstruct your baby's passage down through the pelvis. And perhaps take a couple of your codeine or paracetamol and codeine painkillers.

Remind yourself that every contraction is a step nearer to having your baby. Remember that it is perfectly usual for a first labour to last for 24–48 hours. Although this may sound daunting, reassure yourself that you were designed to be in labour and your body can cope. Of course you will get tired, fed up, will want a break, and be tempted to have any painkillers going, but if you can be patient, your labour will progress.

During the latent stage, your midwife may or may not visit. She knows that you are a mammal and that mammals need privacy and darkness. She also knows that being observed could well stop you labouring so efficiently. So when exactly should you call her?

If any of the following occurs, then it is time to alert your midwife: if your waters break; if you have lost enough blood to fill an egg cup; or if you start mooing!

If your waters break

This is when the bag of membranes lining your uterus pops and some of the amniotic fluid escapes. This can happen at the beginning of labour or even before labour has really started, but usually waters break just before you begin to push your baby out. This is brilliant because it means that just before your baby emerges, your vagina is cleaned by the rush of fluid.

The waters should be clear, pink or mottled, with globs of creamy vernix – the substance that protects your baby's skin from the prolonged immersion in fluid. If your baby is overdue, the waters may also be brown or green. If you can, tell your midwife the colour.

If you lose blood

During labour, any activity can make you lose a small amount of blood. While any spotting or blood loss should be reported to your midwife, it is often completely harmless. (You don't need to call her if you've had blood-stained mucus – the 'show' that appears when the mucus plug that protects your cervix dislodges.)

In pregnancy, the whole genital area is suffused with blood – look at yourself with a mirror and you will see that your genital area is not its usual pink colour, but purple, and this is because there is so much blood coursing through it. So any little effort or scratch can cause bleeding. However, it's best to report any blood loss so your midwife can rule out any condition – such as placental abruption, where the placenta starts to come away from the wall of the uterus – that would require monitoring in hospital.

You start mooing!

What on earth do I mean by, 'when you start mooing'? Remember that childbirth is part of our sex lives. We crave privacy and darkness for both. During sex, we often make noises that we don't normally make. We groan, moan and bellow, and your partner does the same. During labour, with oxytocin coursing through your veins, you may well become aware that there is a funny noise coming in snatches, and then realise that it's coming from you! Mooing, moaning and groaning as you become in tune with your body and the primitive act of childbirth.

The first stage of labour

The first stage of labour is when the uterus is pulling up the cervix. The cervix becomes softer and thins as it is pulled up into the body of the uterus. Then it begins to open, centimetre by centimetre, until it is 10 cms dilated and completely absorbed by the uterus. The uterus has become shorter and thicker and the cervix has become part of the uterine wall, continous with the vagina – one long tunnel, but a very stretchy, soft, loose tunnel, which opens up for the baby. The design is quite magical.

In a first labour, this stage alone can last for 24–48 hours, or even more. Even if it doesn't last that long, it can feel like an eternity. It is a boring, tedious and demanding process for all involved, which takes patience, more patience, and then some.

At the very beginning of labour, most women feel excited. They ring their mum to tell her and they announce it on Facebook. Then they bounce about and wonder when the baby will emerge. As time goes by they become quieter. With the increasing contractions they become stiller. They go into themselves and don't want to talk. They hate being distracted as they concentrate on dealing with each contraction. As they become more and more distant, the partner often starts to feel rather neglected and lonely. Don't worry, she can hear your voice and will appreciate it when you say words of encouragement: 'You are doing well', 'You are dealing with the contractions beautifully', 'Well done darling, the baby is on its way'.

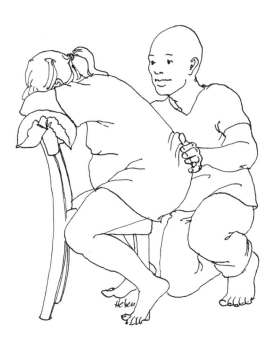

Pain relief during labour

For observers, it is obvious that some contractions during labour are very painful and others are simply very strong sensations. It seems to me that it must be something to do with how your baby is lying, how efficient your uterus is and how peaceful and reassuring your surroundings are. However you're coping, it is reassuring to know that there are therapies and drugs that can help you along the way if you feel the need.

British midwives carry Entonox, commonly known as 'gas and air'. This is an analgesic gas that is a mixture of oxygen, which is good for the baby, and nitrous oxide, which is the analgesic part. Inhaled most commonly through a mouthpiece, gas and air can numb the pain. You need to take at least four deep inhalations before it begins to work. Time your inhalations so that you take them at the start of a contraction; that way you will feel the effects as the contraction peaks.

Some midwives attending homebirths carry pethidine with them, which is an opiate analgesic similar to morphine. It is given as an injection either into your bottom or thigh. It can distance you from the pain, although some women find it makes them feel very fuzzy and out of touch with labour. On the other hand, it can allow you two to three hours' sleep during the latent phase of labour, which can often feel like a frustrating and unproductive stage.

As discussed earlier, warm water is a very effective way to help the management of pain in labour, which is why so many women opt for a birthing pool (see p.32). If you don't have a birthing pool, you can try kneeling on all fours in the shower while the water cascades down your back, or be on all fours in the bath while your partner pours warm water over your back. Some women recline in the bath and sip their drink, others listen to music or their hypno-birthing tapes – do whatever takes your fancy.

Keeping your blood sugar levels high helps the perception of pain, so munch and suck during labour. Your partner's presence and loving stroking can help too, as do their words of encouragement. The midwife saying 'You are doing really really well' also helps you to deal with pain.

Keeping the whole atmosphere upbeat and joyful is very helpful. If there is a lull, a change of scenery can be beneficial – perhaps moving from the bedroom to the sitting room. Generally keeping active is hugely helpful for the progress of labour. If you feel like walking around this is good because the movement can stimulate stronger uterine contractions and shorten your labour. But you may prefer to stay still – it's up to you.

Striding up and down the stairs opens your pelvis and helps to encourage contractions, and going up and down stairs sideways can help to move your baby into a better position for the birth. Don't overdo it though, you may well need energy reserves for later.

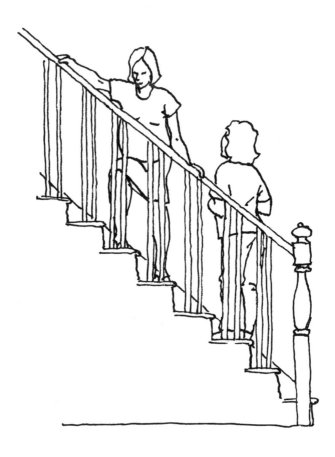

Positions to help manage the pain

If you are at home, one of the bonuses is that you have so many different aids already in place to help you get into different positions: you have work surfaces and window sills to lean against; stairs so you can squat on the bottom step; the lavatory to sit on – back to front is good; a sofa to lean forwards onto; soft flooring to kneel on; walls to rub your back against when it is sore; doors to pull against; and chairs to lean against and to sit on, back to front.

Squatting between your partner's knees can be very helpful in opening your pelvis as fully as possible. However, make sure that they don't leave their arms under your armpits as they could bruise a nerve and disable your arms for the first week of your baby's life. Not to be recommended!

And finally, you and your partner have the privacy to kiss and cuddle and spend time together. All of which will help with your labour, as I explain next.

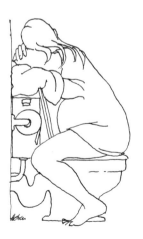

1. On the lavatory
Lavatories are beautifully shaped for comfortable sitting, either the normal way round or back to front. With the added bonus of being able to close the door and ensure privacy. Your partner can stay outside the room or can be with you – stroking your back or kneading your hips – just tell them what you would like.

2. Squatting

This position opens your pelvis beautifully and if you are tired it can be very supportive. Keep an eye on your armpits, don't stay in this position for hours (easily done as it's so comfortable), because the nerves in your axilla (armpits) can get numbed after prolonged time in this position.
So, move around every hour at the very least.

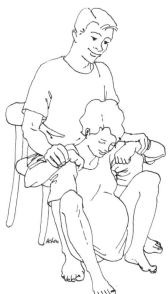

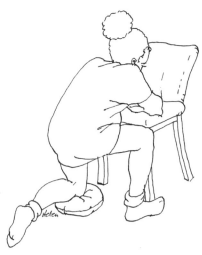

3. Using a chair

In this position, your pelvis is opened up and changed. It gives the baby the opportunity to get into the best position for birth. Try the other leg as well, but it is likely that you will know by instinct which side you need to be working on.

4. Leaning forwards

All of these positions are basically similar and can be done at home or in hospital. Move your pelvis from side to side rhythmically, this opens the pelvis and enables your baby to get into an advantageous position for birth. It also keeps your head above the source of pain, which helps you to manage it better.

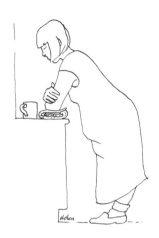

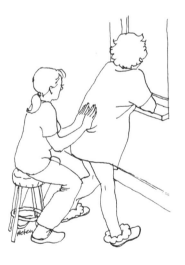

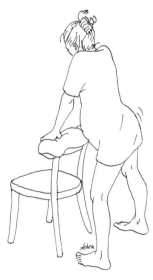

5. The best position of all – especially in hospital

Here you are on all fours between your partner's legs. Your knees are protected from the hard floor. Your partner can cup their hands over your eyes to shield them from the light. You are supported physically by your partner and are surrounded by them. Because of this you can use this position if you are feeling weary, it enables your pelvis to be open and the sacrum and coccyx to flip upwards and out of the way.

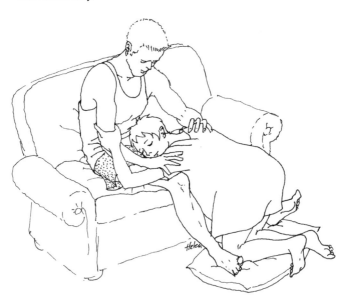

Best of all you can smell your partner, which is a sure way of producing oxytocin. It may sound a bit crude, and we are not like some of our fellow mammals who greet each other by smelling each other's bottoms, we have become much too sophisticated for that! But believe it or not, the scent of your partner, particularly their genitals, is a pleasant aroma for most people and during childbirth will help the labouring woman to produce lots of oxytocin and progress the labour along.

This position is excellent in hospital as long as you can protect your knees from the hard floor. It cuts out all the strangeness of the alien environment and takes you to a very intimate and cosy place surrounded by your partner's smell and touch.

The secret ingredient

That last point brings me to the release of oxytocin. Now you may be embarrassed to hear it, but I'm not embarrassed to say that sexual stimulation is useful during labour. The oxytocin released increases the amount of endorphins you produce and this acts as a natural pain reliever. You may want to be stroked or caressed by your partner – and you can do those in your own home. It's best if the midwife keeps away at this point to give you both privacy!

You will experience many different feelings at this stage of labour. Often women get into the rhythm of the contractions, even dozing in between them.

Throughout labour, you should empty your bladder regularly. You may forget, so it is useful if your partner reminds you now and again, and assists you if you need support.

It can seem as though you have been going on like this for days. A comfortable rhythm of contractions, then relaxing, before surrendering to them again. A manageable process of being a mammal in labour, and then suddenly ... CRASH!

The transitional phase of labour

It may have been okay five minutes ago, but it is definitely not okay now. You are hurting too much, you are fed up to the back teeth, you have had enough. This must stop now. 'Get an ambulance and take me to hospital for an epidural,' you shriek. 'Stop rubbing my back and caressing me.' Whatever your partner is doing is wrong and you hate it.

By now, your midwife should be with you. If she isn't, get your partner to ring her and ask her to come straightaway. She will probably do so quite willingly!

You may be trembling at this stage, you may vomit, you may cry and swear at your partner. Your contractions will be more frequent and more intense. You are at the end of your tether. Hopefully your midwife will say to you, 'This is transition, soon you will be pushing your baby out.' Transition doesn't happen to everyone, but when it does it is quite noticeable.

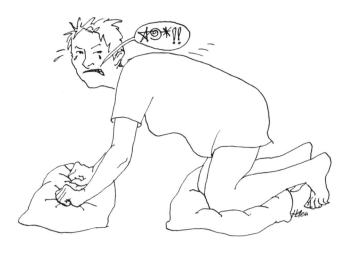

I have looked after my daughter three times in labour and she always says at this stage, 'I can't do this!' When told that she can and that she is doing very, very well, she gets really cross with me. She appeals to her partner to take charge because, as she tells him, 'She knows nothing!' She really hates me at this point because she is feeling overwhelmed – and obviously it is all my fault. Then she begins to grunt, and very soon a beautiful baby will begin to emerge. It is a wonderful moment.

Transition is when everything is too much. But it is also heartening because it is a sign that the second – or pushing – stage of your labour is starting: the stage when your baby is born.

The second stage of labour

Well, several things happen now. Usually this is when your waters break, which is an indication that your cervix is, or is close to being, fully dilated. You feel an urge to push as the baby is beginning to emerge. You will no doubt hear yourself grunting like a child on the potty who goes puce in the face as they push out a poo. Funnily enough, the emerging baby will feel like a big poo, which causes some women concerns.

As a culture, we are rather hung up about faeces. Some women hold back in labour, embarrassed because they feel that they are going to defecate (do a poo) in front of others. Trust me, it is the baby you are feeling. And what's more, holding back is not helpful. The skin between the rectum (back passage) and your vagina is very thin. The baby's head in your vagina presses against the back of your anus and feels like the biggest poo you have ever done.

Now midwives LOVE poo. When they see a tiny bit, they put on their gloves, sweep it up in a tissue and pop it in a bin. But if you watch, they are smiling. They are smiling because you have just shown them that the baby's head is coming down your vagina and everything is progressing well.

The muscles you use to push out your baby also push out any faeces. Rest assured, though, that you are very unlikely to do a huge poo. Most women have diarrhoea before labour starts: this is nature's way of clearing out your back passage. The tiny bit of faeces that comes out in labour is usually no bigger than a walnut. It is important that you don't hold back, so that you push to let your baby out. Relax, and when you have the urge and the midwife tells you, push as hard as you can.

Pushing a first baby out can take up to two to three hours. The pushing contractions come only about every 10 minutes, so you need to push as hard as you can when they do come. For some women it can be frightening and feel dreadful, as though you are going to tear, but this is unlikely. For others, it can be orgasmic. The progesterone of pregnancy has made your vagina softer, looser and stretchier than it has ever been in your life. There is plenty of room – you just need to trust your body, let go and push your baby out.

At the beginning of pushing, women get very excited, as do the midwives and your partner. Something is happening at last, your baby is on the way!

As pushing carries on for an hour, and maybe even approaches two hours, women get despondent: 'It's not coming,' they say. 'It's stuck.' Only when the midwife catches a glimpse of the hair of the baby's head does everyone relax and feel uplifted again.

Then it is really exciting. You can feel the baby coming

– and then going back, and coming again – and going back again. Finally the baby stays there. It doesn't go back any more and the head will soon emerge. Some midwives encourage you to pant rather than push as the head crowns so that the uterus can expel the baby on its own – gently and smoothly with no tearing or trauma.

Your partner needs to be aware that once your baby's head is born it can stay hanging out of the vagina for up to 10 minutes, until the next contraction. During this time, the baby's head becomes rather purple, which is completely normal. With the following contraction, your baby turns and then the whole body emerges quite speedily.

Here is your new baby. If the room is quite dark, they will open their eyes and look at you with interest. If you are lucky, you will fall in love with your baby straightaway. However, it is quite normal not to feel any bond – especially so soon after labour. In Chapter 5, I talk about the gradual bonding process and give you some tips to help you to fall in love with your baby.

The third stage of labour

After your baby's birth, the midwives need to deliver the placenta, or 'afterbirth'. They may use an injection of synthetic oxytocin to encourage your uterus to clamp down and expel the placenta. Or you may prefer to let the umbilical cord carry on pulsating until it stops, and then wait for the placenta to emerge naturally.

There are advantages and disadvantages to both methods. If you have an injection, the whole process is done and dusted in about 20 minutes, and you appear to lose slightly less blood. On the other hand, the concentrated dose of oxytocin can make you feel faint and giddy – although this side effect is quite rare. Also, when the cord is cut before it has stopped pulsating, your baby may have to be helped to start breathing on their own, whereas if you don't have the injection, and wait for nature to take its course, your baby can start to breathe gently and unhurriedly and will get all the blood that they are supposed to from the placenta.

If you take the natural approach, it can take quite a while for the placenta to emerge. During this time you are lying with a cold, clammy umbilical cord protruding from your vagina (I have waited six hours on one occasion). Usually, though, it is out within an hour. If time drags on, you can always ask for the injection.

Interestingly, we are the only mammal that does not eat its placenta. Some women I have known who suffered from bad postnatal depression with a previous pregnancy have frozen their placenta after a subsequent birth, ready to eat if they felt depression coming on. This is not such a mad idea. The placenta is full of hormones and nutrients that are beneficial to the new mother.

Also, some women who have bled very heavily during labour have eaten their placenta and felt immediately regenerated. It can be eaten raw like other mammals do, or cooked. I have cooked it before now for a new mother, served with mashed potatoes and garlic! The revulsion that women feel at the thought of eating it goes immediately when they tuck in. They feel almost miraculously better.

You decide what you want to do. But please don't offer me any!

Moving to hospital

In my experience, first labours are very safe processes. They normally progress slowly, surely and successfully, but it is also true that the women I most commonly transfer from home to hospital are those having first babies. The reason for this has always been that first labours last a long time. Three days, four days, even more. This surely is the time for a lovely epidural and syntocinon (synthetic oxytocin) by intravenous drip to make the contractions more effective and efficient.

The advantage of going to hospital when you are in well-established labour is that no one will send you home saying that you aren't really in labour! Your homebirth midwife may accompany you to the hospital and hand you over to her hospital colleagues, or she may be able to stay with you. It depends on circumstances entirely out of your control.

You may feel buoyed up by the adventure of going in an ambulance and moving to a different location – a change of scene may be exactly what you need. Don't look upon this negatively. Your baby has their own agenda – and this is only the first of many occasions when your plans change because of your children!

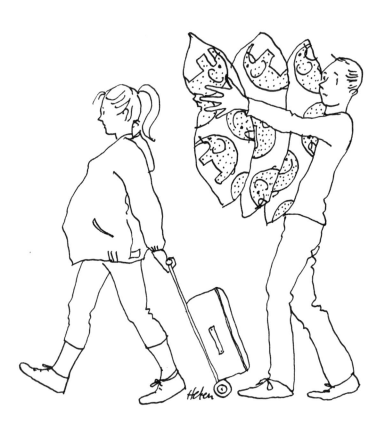

4

Having a homely birth in hospital

You may opt for a hospital birth for several reasons –
perhaps you are being induced because your due date
has long gone and you are still showing no sign of
going into labour naturally. Or you may decide to go
to hospital when your contractions become difficult
to manage. Or you may transfer from home to hospital
because you have been in labour for a long time, you
are exhausted, and your contractions are becoming
less effective.

Whatever your circumstances, no doubt you still like
the idea of having your baby in a comfortable, familiar
environment. So what can you do to make a hospital's
labour ward more home-like? How can you make the room
that you find yourself in 'your home'? It's not easy, but you
can do it.

Think about a hotel room. It isn't really 'your' room,
but you make it your room when you stay there. You might
re-arrange the furniture, spray a scent that you like around
the room, add objects that make it feel more like home –
your laptop, iPad, a framed photograph, even your own
pillow and pillow cases – and no one enters without your
say-so.

The same is true of your room in hospital. Your partner can help to make the room feel like 'your' room, while you are getting on with the business of labour. They can close the blinds or turn the lights off – or down – depending on what sort of lighting there is to make the room darker and more intimate. They can work with the midwife to enable you to move around as much as possible. And if you need to be monitored, they can pull up a chair or birthing ball for you to sit on.

Many hospitals seem to be short of pillows – this is a perfect excuse for you to take in two or three of your own. You will find that these pillows are enormously helpful during labour, and after your baby is born.

Make sure that the pillows have pillow cases that are easily recognisable. Try to avoid white pillow cases, as these may become muddled with hospital ones. Your pillows feel like home, they look like home and they smell like home. You can use them on the bed in the usual way; you can also kneel on them on the hard floor when you are on all fours or lean on them when you are kneeling on the bed in labour; and have them behind you to support your back when you are sitting in an armchair. You will be so glad you took your pillows with you.

Another way that your partner can make the room more homely is by acting as the host. To help get into the mindset for this, they need to think that you have both paid for the room – which of course, you have! In the UK, the whole birthing experience costs about £4,500 (maybe more these days) and you have paid for this out of your taxes and National Insurance contributions.

So, here's your partner, in the room they have paid for, acting as the host. Every time someone comes in, they can open the door with a welcoming smile and outstretched hand and introduce themself, 'Hi, I'm Alex, how do you do?'

After this cue from them, the person will say, 'Oh hello, I'm Doris the domestic, I just need to empty your bin'; or 'I'm Martha the midwife and I need to see if there's a spare blood pressure machine in this room'; or 'I'm Dr Jones and I just wanted to say hello in case you need me later for an epidural.'

While all this is going on you will be in labour, going deep inside yourself and finding it very difficult to be interrupted. Now, instead of having to look up to see who is coming into the room, you can simply listen to the conversation while remaining focused on your contractions. You don't need to join in the conversation. You can be confident that your partner knows you better than anyone else and they can answer for you. 'Of course, come in, Doris!'; 'Thank you, Dr Jones, but we seem to be getting on fine at the moment. Can we come back to you on the epidural if things become more demanding?'

What can you bring to hospital to make it more homely?

So what items can you have in your hospital bag that will help make the room more like home? Some people like to have familiar pictures around them. I have delivered babies while being overlooked by a photo of someone's dog, a photo of someone's deceased mother and a photo of a couple's cottage in the country. A familiar, well-loved photograph can really lift your spirits.

Of course, you won't have access to your food cupboards in hospital, but as before, you will need to keep your strength and sugar levels up. The strong, efficient muscle that is your uterus contracts every 5–10 minutes throughout labour, which over the course of 1–2 days is a lot of contracting. When such an enormous muscle is working so hard, your energy levels are depleted quite quickly. Think about how you normally feel when your blood sugar levels are low: tired, lethargic, shaky, faint, despondent and fed up! When women run on empty during labour, the pain feels much worse than it is. So fill your hospital bag with drinks and snacks to sustain you. Drink squash with your water, suck sweets, chocolate and spoonfuls of honey from the jar, munch on muesli bars – all of these will help you to maintain your blood sugar levels and cope with pain.

Many women find that music really helps them to relax during labour. Whether it's soothing classical music, or pumping rock music – make a playlist and pack your headphones.

Smell is also evocative and helps you create a more familiar environment. While it isn't safe to burn candles in a labour room because of the presence of a large quantity of oxygen, you can spray the room with your favourite scent or room freshener.

The ante- and postnatal wards are generally kept at a very warm temperature, so a small fan is helpful. A flannel is useful too so your partner can wet it with cold water and wipe the back of your neck, your face and your back – helping to keep you as cool and comfortable as possible.

Just as with a homebirth, what you wear to labour in hospital is important. Loose-fitting, comfortable clothing is a must; an old T-shirt and leggings or shorts are perfect. Your partner should also wear light, loose-fitting clothes in the hospital, but they will need something warmer to go home in if they leave the hospital in the early hours of the morning.

Take a change of clothes in case you vomit or your waters break unexpectedly. As at home, flip-flops are ideal to walk around in and are easy to pack.

Birthing partners

You may want to think about whether you would like your mum, sister, or another woman who has given birth, with you in hospital to bring a sense of normality to the scene. She can help when both you and your partner are tired, nip to the hospital shop for chocolate or a sandwich, and stay with you if your partner wants to head out for a bit of fresh air.

If the thought of your mum being there during the actual birth makes you feel embarrassed, just say that you would like her to come but not to be in the room for the birth itself. She will be so pleased to have been asked to help that I'm sure she wouldn't object.

Privacy

And how do you produce lots of oxytocin – the hormone that you produce when you are making love – when you're in hospital with very little privacy! Obviously it will be much harder to be intimate with your partner, but you can try to take advantage of snatched moments. When you find yourselves alone, it is highly beneficial for your partner to arouse you – kissing you, gently playing with your nipples and stroking your clitoris. These simple intimacies produce lots of oxytocin, which encourages contractions, moving labour along.

When a woman in labour produces oxytocin in large quantities, she also produces endorphins (the body's natural morphines), which makes the pain much more manageable. During labour some women go into a trance-like state, relaxed, comfortable, gently moaning and groaning, similar to when making love. Endorphins also make women feel very sleepy, and often women doze between contractions, so time passes gently and constructively. As the hours slip by, this human mammal's body gets on with its job: opening her cervix and pushing out her baby.

Have your say

The midwives and doctors in hospital are very used to women in labour. They are usually extremely kind and patient and give you their full attention; they want the best for you and your baby. They may be busy, but you won't know that. When they are with you, they are just with you. Their commitment is overwhelming. The doctors in obstetrics are used to discussing options in labour with parents-to-be, so they will usually be happy to talk things through with you.

If, however, you are struggling to get on with a particular midwife or doctor in the unit, your partner can leave the room and ask for the supervisor of midwives to be bleeped. One is on duty 24/7 and can try to sort out any problems. Her job is to enable midwives to fulfil their role and to allow you to have as good and safe an experience as possible. You can use her expertise and influence before, during or after labour to ensure you have a positive experience.

In labour, patience usually brings rewards. Most mammals in labour will deliver their baby with no untoward results, just by waiting patiently. So if a caesarean section is mooted or an IV drip, or any other form of intervention to help speed your progress, and you don't feel you are in need of, or ready for, such intervention, you (or preferably your partner) can negotiate.

'Can we hold off until around 4pm, please? We don't feel that we have had enough privacy and peace and quiet to allow Samantha to really get into her labour. A few more hours before intervention would suit us much better.'

'We know that privacy and darkness help labour along, but we have had no time on our own. Could you leave us for a couple of hours so that we can just get into the labour and see what happens?'

Of course, if the intervention is deemed urgent, the staff will let you know and you won't have a choice. Usually, though, they will be happy to hold off for a few more hours, which can often be enough time to enable you to give birth on your own.

On the other hand, you may be utterly fed up and ready to have that caesarean now, this minute, not in half an hour please! Simply play things by ear.

It can be hard to make important decisions under pressure and when in pain. If you and your partner are struggling with what to do, a useful mnemonic is BRAN:

— What are the **Benefits** of this treatment?
— What are the **Risks** of this treatment?
— Are there any **Alternatives** to this treatment?
— What if we do **Nothing** and just wait?

Your midwife or doctor should be able to provide an explanation and guidance to help you reach the right decision.

Your partner's role in summary:

— To take control of the room and welcome everyone who comes in. To find out who they are and what they need.
— Turn out the lights to make the room as dark as possible.
— Encourage you to move around when appropriate.
— Encourage you to make frequent trips to the loo to keep your bladder empty.
— Offer emotional support with loving words, kisses and cuddles.
— Talk you through any breathing and relaxation techniques.
— Keep you nourished with sweet drinks and snacks.
— Help you find comfortable standing, leaning or squatting positions to keep labour progressing.

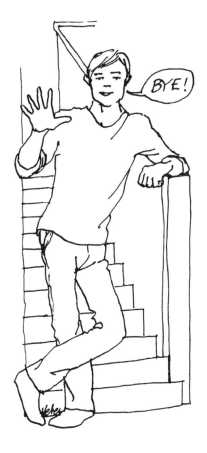

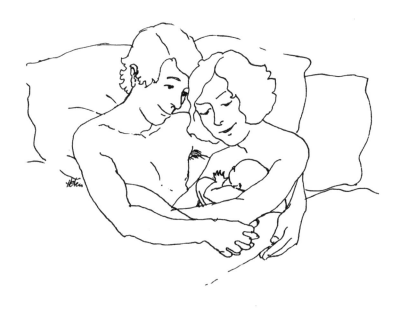

5
Getting to know your baby

Well done, you did it! All the blood, sweat and tears were worth it. Your wonderful new baby is here.

After the birth, the midwives will make sure that you are well. They may help you to have a bath or shower and then they will leave you and your baby in bed together. If you managed to have a homebirth, the very best part can be when the midwives have left. You and your partner can snuggle in your own bed together holding your new baby. You gaze at your baby, you tell each other how clever you both are, you wonder and discuss what happened, you doze and snack, and all the time you are in the bed where you may have conceived this baby. A bed that is comfortable, familiar and comforting. Bliss!

In the first few hours after the birth, you will doze and you will try to feed your baby, which will either go smoothly or not very well. Breastfeeding takes time for you and your baby to work out, and it rarely works well in the first few days. In the next chapter I give some tips on helping you to get started.

In the morning, you will wake up and realise that you have had your baby all night and coped. There is not a manual on how to do this – you are unique and your baby is unique; you are also a mammal and know how to look after your baby. Just try to relax and tune into your instincts. Cats don't go to antenatal classes, sheep don't read parenting guides, elephants, horses and cows all know by instinct how to look after their babies – and so do you. Relax and trust yourself.

A growing bond

So here is the little person you will be spending so much time with, now and for the rest of your life. How do you feel about this person?

If you are very lucky (and very unusual), you may fall in love instantly with your baby. You will recognise their smell, their little round head will feel familiar and their mewling and suckling will be instantly recognisable and lovable.

Yet most women don't fall in love with their baby at first: for many women, love is an emotion that grows over time. The startling thing about babies is that they are people, and when your person is handed to you, or you pick them up for the first time, they may be somebody that you don't take to straightaway. You may be interested in them or intrigued, but feel no 'bond'. Some women say that it's as if the midwife has a bucket of babies next to her and she has picked this one out for you. It's quite a nice baby, but you do not recognise it.

Sadly, some women positively dislike their baby after the birth. They may find them ugly, their cry horrendous, their nose huge – nothing like the little pink-lipped beauty they were expecting. Tired and deflated after the birth, they can feel incredibly disappointed. They may feel that they have made a huge mistake, and the burden of the responsibility they have let themselves in for feels overwhelmingly heavy.

Let's find some ways to help you fall in love with your baby more quickly. You will, of course, fall in love with them eventually, but for some of us it can take weeks. These weeks can seem long and unhappy. So are there any tricks to help you fall in love?

You fall in love with your baby in exactly the same way you fell in love with your partner. At the age of 35, my husband was a confirmed and very shy bachelor. One day he went to a wedding. He heard a clatter at the back of the church and turned round to see what had caused it. He saw the woman he immediately recognised as his future wife, the woman he had been waiting 35 years to meet; he was overjoyed and immediately leapt into action trying to woo her and convince her that he was the man for her. He fell in love at first sight.

I, of course, went to the same wedding. I noticed no one in particular. I greeted my Auntie Freda and my cousins, sat with my sisters and parents, and enjoyed the wedding. At the wedding breakfast I was seated next to this extraordinarily awkward man. His conversation was laboured and rather dull, and he was incredibly shy. He found out that I was coming to London to start my midwifery training. He found out where I would be staying, the hospital where I'd be working. After the wedding breakfast, he asked my dad for a lift back into town. I went home with Auntie Freda after telling my mum that I would not sit in the same car as that revolting man.

From the minute I set foot in London the barrage began: letters, phone calls, theatre tickets, meals out, trips to the cinema. Every time I looked round Giles Flint was there! We got engaged after three months and married seven months later. We have had an extraordinarily blessed marriage for 59 years. I discovered the funniest, kindest, cleverest and most interesting man who has enhanced my life beyond all imagination. I fell in love with him gradually, and surprised myself when I recognised that this was the emotion I felt after a few weeks of going out together.

So how did I fall in love with him? What mechanisms were in place to enable that to happen? And do those same mechanisms help a mother to fall in love with her baby?

Look at people in the first flush of love – what do they do? They gaze at each other, they have eyes only for each other. This also works for you and your baby. You need to gaze at your baby, to get to know every little crease, every aspect of their body, every squeak and sound, every coo and cry.

The other thing that you need to do is to smell your baby. They have a completely unique smell, which is one of the reasons why midwives no longer bath babies when they are very new. The smell of your baby is necessary for you. Think of the people and things you love and their particular smell: your partner, mother, your home. We are mammals, and mammals have a strong and evocative sense of smell.

Babies are designed to help us to fall in love with them: they have big floppy heads and large eyes, which pull at our heartstrings. Moreover, your baby's smell is beautiful, and once they smile, you will automatically fall in love with them. Most babies do not smile for about six weeks, so if you can get your baby to smile earlier, your love will come sooner. The way to get them to smile as early as possible is to talk to them.

Your voice is your baby's favourite sound. While they were in the womb, they heard it all the time. They recognise it instantly and feel cheered and comforted by it, so talk to them all the time. You can talk about your family; you can discuss the news with your baby; or the cricket or football; and you can give your opinion on the garden, weather and politics. In fact, your baby will be the best listener you have ever had! When you run out of discussion topics, you can also sing to them. The more they hear you, the sooner they will smile at you, and this will strengthen your bond.

So to help you fall in love with your baby as quickly as possible, gaze at them; smell them and talk to them.

Finally, when we are naked we produce the hormone oxytocin – the hormone of love. So lie with your baby and let them be naked next to you, skin to skin: such soft, sweet-smelling skin next to yours.

Or have a bath together in warm, not hot, water: wonderfully calming and soothing for both of you.

The first two weeks

Most partners have two weeks' paternity leave and I would like to suggest that this 10–14 days is taken up with looking after you, the new mum.

Childbirth is an ordeal. However lovely, fulfilling or even orgasmic a birth is, most women are left feeling very stiff and full of aches and pains. If your birth was a ghastly ordeal, you may feel shocked, bruised and may even have flashbacks and frightening dreams. Whatever sort of birth you had, your body will probably feel pretty pummelled and is undergoing huge changes.

Your centre of gravity changes enormously during labour itself. From having a huge uterus that hangs forward, it now shrinks back and your centre of balance shifts. After birth, your body expels all the extra fluids it retained in the blood and tissues during pregnancy, so you will need to visit the lavatory frequently to empty your bladder.

Your breasts start to lactate and change, swelling and developing as they feed your baby. The activity that is going on in your body is greater than when you were going through puberty.

With such monumental changes occurring, it is important to get some rest. For your equilibrium's sake and for your body to heal and regenerate, lie down on a bed to recuperate.

This rest time will allow you to reflect on what has happened to you and how the labour and birth went. Talk with your partner too and discuss what happened when, how the midwife coped with this or that situation, and how you both managed certain parts of your labour. You need to talk through your labour over and over again for it to become part of you and your psyche.

So staying in bed and allowing yourself to be looked after is important to help women recover both mentally and physically. During childbirth, women go through a life-changing experience, more enormous and shocking than they ever envisaged. Labour can go on for longer than imagined and be stronger and more demanding than anyone anticipated, leaving women shaken, exhausted and overwhelmed with the huge responsibility of a new baby. Now you need to be loved, cherished and looked after. There also needs to be an acknowledgement of the huge experience you have dealt with. The easiest and best way to do this is for your beloved partner to look after you and encourage you to stay in bed and luxuriate for the first two weeks, as if you were in a spa or luxury hotel.

The other reason for staying in bed for the first two weeks is to do with your baby.

Your baby wants to communicate with you. When you watch them, they will try to meet your gaze, and react to your every word. Even in the first hours of life they are trying to tell you what they think about the world or what they really want. You will never see this if your baby is stuck in a corner in a Moses basket. They need to be within 12 inches (30 cm) of your face to be able to see you properly. Skin to skin, gazing at each other, smelling each other, talking to each other – you are laying the foundations of one of the most important relationships in both your lives.

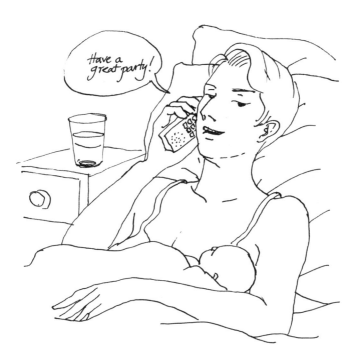

If you have, or had, difficulties with your own mother, remember that this is where your relationship started. You have within you the means to make this a mutually satisfying and loving relationship. Don't waste this precious time doing your emails or chatting on the phone. Shut out the world for a couple of weeks and let your partner look after you. If you don't have a partner, or they can't be around, before your baby is born try and arrange for your mum or a close friend to come and look after you so that you can spend 10 days in bed with your baby. You need someone there who will cook for you, shop for you, do the washing and ironing, and keep the house clean and in order. It is really, really important.

Your recovery

One of the most important things that you can do to help your body regain its shape and suppleness is pelvic floor exercises. It is best to start practising these during pregnancy so that you are able to relax your pelvic floor muscles during the birth. You learn how to contract the muscles of your pelvic floor by going to the lavatory and passing urine. As the urine flows, try to stop it by squeezing the muscles in your genital area. Sometimes you can't actually stop it, but usually you can slow it down. What you have done is identify your pelvic floor muscles. Once you've identified these very important muscles, you then set about exercising them, squeezing the muscles up to 50 times a day – tighten, loosen, tighten, loosen, tighten, loosen, again and again.

When you exercise these muscles after the birth, you help the blood to circulate in that area and so promote healing. By tightening and loosening, you also enable the muscles to become stronger and more springy – which helps enormously when you start making love again, and can prevent problems in later life such as prolapses and incontinence. You can practise these exercises subtly when you are standing in the kitchen, waiting for a bus, peeling potatoes, lying or sitting and feeding your baby – tighten, loosen, tighten, loosen. As a woman who has had a baby, it needs to become a regular part of your life.

After the birth, you also need to keep the genital area very clean, so have a bath every day and gently cleanse all the nooks and crannies. Some herbal products have healing properties, such as Badedas bath gel, which contains horse chestnuts. This is lovely and can be obtained online or from traditional chemists and some supermarkets.

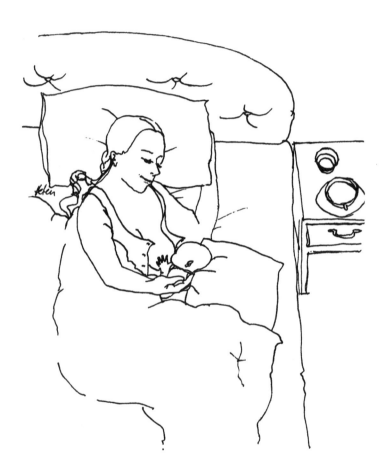

6
Take it easy

You have done the hard work – now the harder work begins!

Breastfeeding is natural and all mammals do it. So it is ridiculous that it can be so difficult: so sore, so demanding, so inscrutable, so undermining.

This is yet another reason to stay in bed for up to two weeks after the birth. Being close to your baby enables breastfeeding to happen and to work. Your baby needs to be close to the source of food, to smell you and instinctively turn and root for your nipple. With you observing your baby, you will learn to read their cues and what they are trying to tell you. They will be saying things to you moments after the birth: babies are outrageously opinionated!

One of the best ways to breastfeed is to lie on your side. This means that your baby is also on their side. Their tummy is against your body and their mouth can reach your nipple and areola (the area around your nipple). Your baby's head is as wide as their shoulders, so they don't need a pillow – they can suckle from either breast depending on what your shape is like. Some women manage best with the lower breast nearest to the baby; women with softer breasts may prefer to use their upper breast. Breastfeeding on your side initially avoids putting pressure on your sore genital area, especially sensitive if you had stitches; and if you had a caesarean, being on your side stops your baby pressing on your tummy. You can also doze while feeding them (being a mammal, instinctively you won't lie on them).

The more you feed your baby, the easier it will become. As your baby grows, their mouth grows and it is easier for them to latch on to your breast. Also, as they grow, they take more milk into their stomach and go longer between feeds.

It is a very clever supply and demand system: your baby's sucking triggers the release of hormones that signal your body to produce milk to their exact requirements. So if your baby sucks more, you produce more milk. If you had twins and have two babies who are both suckling from you, you will produce enough milk for two babies.

Women often fear that they do not have enough milk. If you really feel that you are not producing enough milk, you may not be resting enough. When you are on night duty, being woken several times during the night, it is essential to get at least two hours' rest during the day. You can always find an opportunity to rest when your baby is sleeping. Ideally lie down on your bed, with your baby if you like, rather than doze on a sofa.

So, you are looking after yourself and resting during the day, all of which helps you to produce milk and breastfeed. Drink lots of water to rehydrate you and eat as well as you can – cake is a lovely indulgence for breastfeeding mothers – and have nutritious snacks on hand to keep your energy levels up.

For the first two weeks, having your baby clamp on to your breast can make your nipples very sore. If you do feel discomfort or pain, this should pass by the time you've counted to 15. After the first two weeks, this sensation should go as your nipples become acclimatised to breastfeeding. Many books say that if breastfeeding hurts then you are doing it incorrectly. This seems wrong to me. Our nipples are one of the most sensitive areas of our anatomy. They are used to being treated with love and respect – not being attacked every hour and a half. No wonder they are sore!

If you are worried about your technique or struggling to feed, ask your midwife, local NCT breastfeeding counsellor or contact the La Leche League who can all help (see 'Resources' at the end of the book).

Breastfeeding support cafes, often set up by local hospitals, can provide a safe and comfortable environment to support breastfeeding women so ask your midwife or health visitor if there's one nearby. Here you can meet up with other new mums for a cup of tea and have a breastfeeding expert on hand to help you with feeding. There are also places to ring where you can get advice and support, so do reach out if you are struggling.

Visitors

You will be amazed at how popular you become once you have had a new baby. Other people are fascinated by babies and all sorts will beat a path to your door: people you used to work with but haven't seen for years; your old next-door neighbour; someone from the local church; the lady at the corner shop who sells you your newspaper. They will all come – all bearing gifts, some appropriate, some not. So what if it gets a bit much?

You need to work out a strategy for visitors. You could decree family and close friends only for the first two weeks. Or maybe no visitors at all for the first 10 days, or all visitors between 2–4 pm on Sundays. Find what feels comfortable for you, your partner and your baby.

Remind yourself that you are a mammal and that baby mammals need to be in close proximity to their mother. So your baby needs to be kept close to you. Once your baby has been handed round the room and jiggled and distracted, they will come back to you feeling disorientated and upset. They will also smell differently. Instead of smelling like your baby, they will smell of Chanel No 5 or coffee.

So even though visitors are well meaning, their presence can sometimes do more harm than good at this early stage. While they may bring food and help out, they will distract you from your breastfeeding project. You may be embarrassed to feed the baby in front of Uncle Joe, your father-in-law, your brothers – anyone really. Their bustle can exhaust you in your vulnerable and sensitive state. And they will all have lots of advice, whether or not they have had a baby of their own, which can overwhelm and confuse you.

Try and avoid entertaining visitors in the main living room – your partner can do this while you stay in bed. Visitors can then come into the bedroom in small groups to see you and the baby. Make sure that your partner clears them out quite quickly though!

If your partner serves tea and coffee in the sitting room, they can usually lure people back there. Under no circumstances allow your baby to go down and be passed around. The poor little thing will be completely muddled and confused; they need to be quiet and snuggled up to you. Your baby's world has been you all their life. Your uterus has cuddled them constantly since they were conceived and your body has fed them constantly. All they have ever heard has been your voice, your heartbeat, you singing, shouting, talking to your partner, your music, your TV programmes.

The stimulus of lots of visitors can be too much for a very new baby. They need to be next to you and safe from noise, excitement, other people's smells and rough fabrics.

And it can also be too much for you. Getting to know your baby, learning what they are saying to you and learning to breast or bottle-feed will take all your time during the first couple of weeks. You do not have the time to be a gracious hostess, nor do you have the energy – escape to your bed, to your sanctuary.

When you don't feel right

We don't exactly know what causes postnatal depression – it could be hormonal, it could be physical, or it could just be that you are exhausted with the demands of a small baby. I believe firmly that our culture makes it very hard to be the mother of a small baby. There is sometimes a competitiveness among women and you may overhear them saying things like:

'I did a big supermarket shop two days after my caesarean.'

'My baby slept through the night from eight days.'

'Oh, she's been sitting up for ages!'

I've even heard people in my own profession saying things like:

'Childbirth is a natural process, now just get on with your life.'

'Don't lie in bed, you'll get deep vein thrombosis.'

Having a baby is completely life-changing. There is before birth and there is after birth – they are two different countries. And just like moving to a new country, you have to learn the language and how they do things: it takes time and effort.

During childbirth, your body has taken a physical battering. It feels pummelled and disorientated. If your labour was a long, drawn-out process, you will be feeling exhausted. In the early days and weeks, you can feel that you never catch up on the sleep you have lost, and find it impossible to get on top of things. You may just about get through the day.

Emotionally things have been done to your body that may feel shocking and intrusive. The numerous internal examinations, however gentle, can still feel invasive and demeaning. If you had forceps, a ventouse or a caesarean, you may get flashbacks and feelings of distress – which is to be expected when your body has been invaded, albeit beneficially.

So after the initial euphoria of producing a happy, healthy baby subsides, you may start to feel numb, disorganised and unable to get things done. What can you do to start feeling like your old self again?

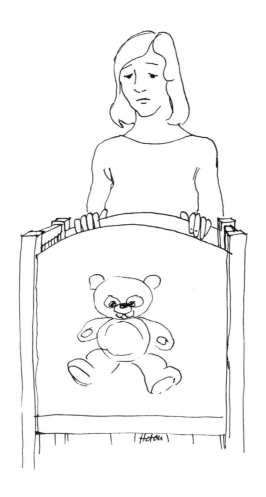

Depression is not a very useful name for feeling like this, but if you imagine all your systems being depressed – not quite working properly – you can see why your brain is unusually slow and ponderous, your walking is slow and your legs are heavy, why everything is such a huge chore.

I feel deeply that it is important for women to acknowledge all the physical and emotional changes they've experienced. This is why I suggest that after the birth you look after yourself – in fact convalesce as if you've had a major operation (you will be more likely to do this if you had a caesarean section, but still do it even if you had a very gentle natural birth). When you convalesce, you rest your body, giving it a chance to heal and recuperate, and giving yourself a chance to think through the labour. As we discussed earlier, resting while being looked after also gives you the opportunity to get to know your baby and for the two of you to learn to breastfeed. Being cherished and cared for may be enough to nip any lurking postnatal depression in the bud.

You will also adapt to your baby's pattern of sleeping, which can be challenging after a lifetime of eight hours' sleep a night. New babies sleep roughly for an hour and a half and then wake for a feed, then they sleep for two hours and wake for a feed, then they sleep for an hour and three-quarters and wake for a feed – and so it goes on. By staying in bed with your baby you will adapt to their natural rhythm and learn to 'nap'.

Following this lovely, gentle time with your newborn baby, it is important for you to factor resting into your life in these first months. You should rest on your bed for 1–2 hours every day, rain or shine, while your baby naps. If you find that your mind is too busy, don't fret – have a radio in your room and listen to programmes or plays, or to music. Relaxing to lovely music is one of the most healing and beautiful things that you can do for yourself.

Think about women in India where they have a deep respect and acknowledgement of women who have just had a baby. For six weeks (40 days), the woman has a daily massage (as does the baby). She is given healing and nourishing foods and nothing is expected of her. She doesn't cook, she doesn't get ready to go out – she stays indoors and simply looks after the baby and rests. It is acknowledged that she is to be cherished and cared for. She is 'special' – as are you at this time.

Of course, if you do feel that you have succumbed to postnatal depression, please do go to your doctor who can prescribe some effective anti-depressants. Within a couple of weeks you should feel better and the clouds lift. Often you need to take them for a few months and then see how you are getting on.

Postnatal depression usually lasts until the baby is about a year old and then it lifts – often never to return again. I had postnatal depression after my second child. I woke every morning dreading the day, was foul to my husband and little son, grumpy, barking and irritable. I couldn't function properly, life was too much. When the baby was a year old, I was transformed into my usual bubbly self – active, eager, bossy and full of beans. When I was expecting my third child I was very afraid that I would suffer again – but no, after his birth I felt fabulous and competent. Extraordinary.

As well as anti-depressants, walking and talking can help enormously too!

Once you get your strength back, walking briskly will get your hormones flowing and lift your spirits. Aim to go out every day – walk in the park, or to a mothers' coffee group or baby massage group. You need to see and talk to other people, and gradually you will feel better.

Counselling can make a significant difference to postnatal depression. If you can find yourself a good counsellor, they can help you to move along and feel much better. Your doctor may have a counsellor in the practice whom you can access. Counselling doesn't change the way you do things, but it speeds the process of recovery and enables you to regain strength and heal more quickly.

Good luck. I am actually eternally grateful that I had postnatal depression. It increased my knowledge and understanding of other human beings. It made me less arrogant, more humane and less judgemental. It has been very useful in my work, although it was foul at the time.

7
My dream

Well, my nightmare is that childbirth here is becoming more like it is in Brazil which has one of the highest rates of caesareans in the world: 55 per cent of all deliveries, up to 85 per cent in private hospitals (compared to 32 per cent in the US and 29 per cent in the UK). Does it matter, you might ask. I think it does.

An elective caesarean is quite a nice way of having a baby: the mother is conscious and ready to greet her baby; the partner can plan to be off work and at the birth. It is convenient because we know the intended day and time, so can plan accordingly. Your mum can travel up to be there, everything can be ready. It's rather like booking a holiday – all sorted. It is all so much more civilised than the sweaty, puking and passionate process that is natural birth.

Of course, you may not have a choice in the matter, but this rosy picture leaves out a few uncomfortable facts about caesareans: how some women experience pain afterwards for several months, or the increased risks with a second birth (such as retained placenta or uterine rupture). And what about the overhang of abdominal skin that distresses women once their scar has healed. Or the extra exhaustion felt by a woman who has lost more blood than in a normal birth. It has to be said, though, that many women appear to manage well after a caesarean section and are happy with them.

However, something in me feels that the passionate, heaving, moaning intensity of a normal birth is there for a purpose. That the endorphins released during labour are produced, in part, to enable the love we feel towards our babies. Maybe it's just me, but I love a bit of passion and emotion.

In my dream, there isn't a hospital because, in my opinion, all women with straightforward pregnancies would fare better if they stayed at home with a nice midwife and were able to transfer to hospital if they needed to. The closest I came to achieving my dream was during the 22 years that I ran my birth centre in London. Here I tried to provide the perfect place and environment for women to labour and give birth.

The ideal place for a couple to have their baby would be reminiscent of a hotel where they would book into their room. They would be greeted by a doula or a kindly (probably older) woman who would be available to them throughout her shift. The room would be comfortable, clean and fragrant. There would be a large sofa bed with space for parents and the baby. The room would have very dark blinds so it could be completely blacked out if desired, and there would be music of choice, and refreshments in the fridge with extra space for the couple to bring the things they like to eat and drink. The bedroom door would lock and there would be no clock. No one would enter without being checked out first by the parent-to-be.

In the corner would be a deep birthing pool – already

filled with water at the right temperature. The floors would be soft so that kneeling for many hours would be possible. In our birth centre, over the whole 22 years we had only one woman who gave birth lying on the bed – everyone else chose to be kneeling, standing, squatting, anything but lying on their backs.

I envisage one or two midwives who are in charge of the safety of the mothers and babies. So, on arrival, the midwife would come into the room, greet the couple and explain what is expected of them and check out the mother and baby. She would check the mother's temperature, pulse and blood pressure, and do a urine analysis and abdominal palpation. She would also check the baby's position and presentation, how far she was engaged, and would keep an eye on the fetal heart rate and whether the waters had broken.

I wouldn't expect a vaginal examination to be carried out unless it was absolutely necessary. The midwife should be able to tell if the mum-to-be is in established labour and how far she has progressed.

The couple would be told that they will be left on their own unless they ring the buzzer. The partner's role is to seduce their partner, to love her, to stroke her, to kiss her – to generally make out. They can get undressed, gambol in the pool or on the soft floor or sofa, loving and playing with each other.

I understand for many readers that 'making love to order' can be off-putting. That women may feel timid at the thought that people might know what is going on! But I envisage that appealing to the partner might make them much more receptive, and if they know that all this foreplay can result in the safe birth of their child, and if they are assured that no one can come in without them opening the door, we could rely on them more to get things going.

During early labour, the fetal heart rate needs to be listened to rarely: only when the strongly contracting uterus is putting pressure on the baby's head is the baby at any kind of risk, and usually not even then. Human mammals are beautifully designed to produce their babies gently and safely.

There will be long labours and demanding labours, but most will be manageable.

One of the ways for women to feel free to labour for a long time is by remaining at home, ideally with a midwife visiting, at least until they are in established labour. One of the most wasteful aspects of maternity hospitals is the number of women who occupy wards when they are not really in labour. Many hospitals try to overcome this with a 'triage' nurse, who assesses a woman on arrival and either gives her a bed or sends her home and tells her to come back later.

In my dream, there would be delivery suites as there are now, where doctors can intervene if there is a medical reason to. However, there would be very few of them because if you leave women alone to get on with their labour – like other mammals – they usually manage to give birth safely.

The only reason that my dream is unlikely to ever take off is because it would involve people losing jobs. The need for so many doctors would drop phenomenally, fewer obstetricians would be needed, fewer anaesthetists and fewer paediatricians. The number of midwives would not drop substantially, nor would it rise. They would be supervising the doulas who would be doing the comforting, encouragement and general succour of women and their partners.

The costs of the maternity services would probably

halve, which is the only reason I ever have to be hopeful that my dream might come true. The cost of caesarean sections is prohibitive – maybe price will be the defining factor that will enable women to have better births!

Midwives in this country are very well trained and knowledgeable and their practical experience is excellent. Their only handicap at the moment is that they are intimidated by guidelines and policies, by so many of their profession having become institutionalised, and a very punitive philosophy. Midwives need to be given the freedom to practise as they know best, and to be given professional managers – people who know how to lead and inspire – rather than midwives who have risen to the top without adequate management training.

There are, of course, some midwifery managers who have natural management skills. In my local hospital, midwives who were despondent and aggrieved are now motivated and engaged because of a gentle and encouraging Head of Midwifery.

When enabled and encouraged to work to their best levels, midwives are absolutely wonderful. Their love of women and the miraculous process of birth means they can thrive in the right environment and become addicted to the profession.

Midwifery is a job, but it is also a very real vocation. That is why in any hospital you will see midwives who look as if they should have retired long ago. It is simply because being present when a woman gives birth is one of life's greatest fascinations. Seeing a woman empowered and drawing from her deepest reserves during labour is incredible. And seeing the tenderness of their partner towards them and their newborn baby is beautiful.

Almost all women feel nervous before they go into labour. Will it be too painful? Will I be able to manage? Will my partner be frightened? Be aware that you are a mammal, that human mammals have been giving birth since the dawn of time. Your mother, your grandmother, your great-great-grandmother all gave birth. And so will you.

When labour begins, often women relax because in many ways it feels familiar. 'Oh yes,' they say, 'this is not new and frightening. I've done this before, I have been here before.' And the birth that follows is a completely miraculous and magical experience. It stays with you forever and, like those strong female ancestors before you, it will define you and become part of your life story.

And, of course, the birth will become the opening chapter in your child's own story.

Being a midwife is a privilege and a huge pleasure. It's like witnessing a small miracle on a daily basis. To see a nervous young woman become a proficient mother – and an intimidated partner become a skilful parent – is such a wondrous and enjoyable experience. And having a baby is the most life-changing, life-enhancing and demanding experience we ever go through. I hope this little book will help a bit – a friend with you on your way, on this the most exciting adventure of your lives.

Common questions

Q. Isn't it dangerous to have a baby at home?

A. Not at all. Research has consistently shown that childbirth at home is a very safe option. Take a look yourself by visiting: *cochrane.org* (then search under 'childbirth at home')

––––––––––

Q. Surely it must be better to be in hospital because the right equipment and staff are on hand if anything goes wrong?

A. The disadvantage of having so much stuff there – in case anything goes wrong – is that it tends to be over-used. Equipment like electronic fetal heart monitors is very expensive and needs to be used to justify its purchase. Ultrasound scans have never been shown by research to be of any real clinical benefit – most things like twins or placenta praevia can be diagnosed with palpation (when a midwife or doctor feels the abdomen), as was the case before scans came on the scene – yet every woman seems to have several scans during pregnancy, costing the country a fortune.

Women are also very susceptible to atmosphere while in labour and if they are in an environment where people are consistently thinking 'We're here just in case something goes wrong, just in case an emergency happens', it makes emergencies much more likely to happen.

In my experience (working in a town with a very good ambulance service), virtually any emergency can be dealt with speedily by a midwife at your home informing the hospital that she is on her way with that particular emergency. The staff in the labour ward react and prepare appropriately for the admission and any situation is dealt with swiftly and efficiently when you arrive.

With first-time mothers, the most usual reason to transfer is because the labour has been going on for days and everyone is fed up, tired and needing some help with moving the labour along.

Q. Isn't homebirth really messy? I wouldn't want to be clearing up blood-stained sheets and towels after I had given birth.

A. Midwives are enormously practical. They bring large, absorbent sheets that they lay over the floor. Most midwives would be mortified to think that they had left any trace of blood in your home. They pride themselves on leaving the birthing room unmarked.

Q. Would a birthing pool be safe in our flat – we are on the third floor. I don't want the ceiling below caving in!

A. Put your pool in the corner of the room – this is the strongest part of a room where the joists cross over each other. Push the empty pool right into the corner before you fill it.

———————

Q. Would it be worth having a doula at our birth?

A. Absolutely. Look up *cochrane.org*, which will show you that having a doula with you increases your chances of having a natural birth, and helps you avoid unnecessary interventions.

If you can't afford a doula, what about asking your mum, a sister or friend. Another woman, as well as your partner, is often very helpful. It brings a normality to the proceedings and a fresh perspective. It means that your partner is supported as well as you.

Resources

Supportive organisations

The NCT
(National Childbirth Trust)
Support line (UK)
0300 330 0700
nct.org.uk
The UK's largest and
most effective charity for
pregnant people. Offers
birth preparation classes,
postnatal groups and
'Walk and Talk' groups
for new parents. Acts as a
mouthpiece for those going
through pregnancy, labour
and childbirth. Evidence-
based information.

—

AIMS
(Association for
Improvements in the
Maternity Services)
Advice line (UK)
0300 365 0663
aims.org.uk
Set up to 'support women
and families to achieve the
birth that they wanted',
AIMS campaigns for
improvements to the UK's
maternity services, offers a
helpline, web resources and
guidebooks.

—

Birthrights
birthrights.org.uk
Champion respectful
care during pregnancy
and childbirth by
protecting human rights.
They provide advice and
information on your legal
rights in childbirth, train
doctors and midwives,
and campaign to change
maternity policy and
systems.

—

Make Birth Better
makebirthbetter.org
Another organisation to
turn to when you need
help and support during
pregnancy and childbirth.

Breastfeeding help

National Childbirth Trust
Feeding Line (UK)
0300 330 0700
A free support line for help with feeding – real humans will talk with you.

—

La Leche League (UK)
0345 1202918
A free support line with access to real humans. Local groups which can be very supportive.

—

Lactation Consultants
Search *'local Lactation Consultant'*. They will come to your home, sort out your problems; most are self-employed but their charges are usually reasonable.

Podcasts/radio

The Obs Pod
The podcast of Florence, an NHS obstetrician on all things maternity related. Interesting, amusing and informative. My favourite episodes are interviews with 'Mr ObsPod' and her fascinating take on homebirths. She works in Kingston, Surrey, where they have one of the best homebirth services in the UK.

—

Woman's Hour
Occasionally has good debates on childbirth. Podcast and BBC Radio 4.

—

The Midwives' Cauldron
Katie James and Dr Rachel Reed discuss midwifery, birth, lactation and womanhood.

Facebook

Home Birth Support Group UK
Source of some fascinating birth stories.

—

Dr Sara Wickham
Sara is an experienced midwife who sifts all the evidence to help you to work out what is safest and best for you. She sends out regular updates to her subscribers. Her books include *In Your Own Time*, about induction of labour; *What's right for me? How to make decisions which suit you* and other recommended publications.
sarawickham.com

—

Biomechanics for Birth
Developed by midwife Molly O'Brien, this applies 'biomechanics', the study of human movement, to childbirth. Includes ways to help the body to be flexible during labour.
optimalbirth.co.uk

Instagram

@kemibirthjoyjohnson
@doulacally
@stockportbirth
@my_expertmidwife
@james_the_midwife
@becwallisbirthkeeper

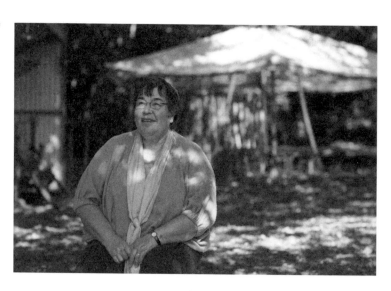

About the author

When I was eight years old, my mother had her fourth baby at home. I can still smell that lovely baby smell, see the red, angry, little face, remember the feel of that soft skin. I knew immediately that I wanted to be a midwife – and that I wanted to have babies of my own. How lucky I've been to have managed both.

I have been a midwife for nearly 50 years working in hospitals, women's homes and The Birth Centre in London that I ran for 22 years. This wonderful place specialised in one-on-one midwifery care with dark, peaceful birthing rooms and a midwifery team who treated birth as a positive, normal, physiological process.

As a mother, I have had three babies at home and managed to breastfeed them. I've watched them all grow up to be such lovely parents themselves and, most wonderfully, I was able to be the midwife at the births of nine of my 12 grandchildren.

I was President of the Royal College of Midwives, a founder member of the Association of Radical Midwives and the first chair of the Midwives Information and Resource Service. I continue to speak at conferences, and run a twice-weekly 'Bumps and Babies' group for the NCT. You can find me on TikTok @carolineflint.midwife.

Thanks

My biggest thank you, as ever, is to Giles Flint who has supported and loved me through thick and thin. He has also been my financial supporter and it was his help that enabled The Birth Centre to function for 22 years.

Thank you to the hundreds of women who have given me the great honour and pleasure to be with them during the births of their babies. They have taught me so much and shown me how magnificent the human mammal is at giving birth.

Thank you to my mother who showed me the wonders of birth when she gave birth to my little sister at home and set me on the path to midwifery. Also her sensible and undramatic attitude to birth helped me when I was expecting my first (and subsequent babies). Her words 'You are never sent more pain than you can bear' rang in my ears while in labour.

Thank you to the hundreds of women and men who have been to my NCT classes. They have made me laugh, they have challenged me, they have helped at nearly-new sales – the taller men have even put up hanging baskets or changed light bulbs when I couldn't reach.

Thank you to my colleagues – especially those who worked with me at The Birth Centre over so many years. Laughter, hugs and wisdom just about sums up my memories of you all.

Thank you to Miranda West at Do Books without whose support and encouragement this book would never have been written.

To Helen Chown who has been drawing women in labour for me and for the NCT for so many years – thank you.

Index

Books in the series

Also available

Available in print, digital and audio formats from booksellers or via our website: **thedobook.co**

To hear about events and forthcoming titles, find us on social media **@dobookco**, or subscribe to our newsletter